Acquisitions Editor: Frances DeStefano
Product Manager: Julia Seto
Senior Manufacturing Manager: Benjamin Rivera
Marketing Manager: Kimberly Schonberger
Director of Creative Services: Doug Smock
Production Service: Aptara, Inc.

Library of Congress Cataloging-in-Publication Data

Lippincott's focus on cardiovascular disease and sleep apnea.
    p. ; cm.
  Adapted from: Handbook of sleep medicine / Alon Y. Avidan, Phyllis C.
Zee. 2006, Fundamentals of sleep technology / Nic Butkov, Teofilo
Lee-Chiong. 2007, and Clinical sleep disorders / Paul R. Carney, Richard
B. Berry, James D. Geyer. 2005.
  Includes bibliographical references.
  ISBN 978-1-60913-005-3
  1. Sleep apnea syndromes. 2. Heart—Diseases—Risk factors. I.
Avidan, Alon Y. Handbook of sleep medicine. II. Butkov, Nic.
Fundamentals of sleep technology. III. Carney, Paul R. Clinical sleep
disorders. IV. Lippincott Williams & Wilkins. V. Title: Focus on
cardiovascular disease and sleep apnea.
  [DNLM: 1. Sleep Apnea Syndromes—complications. 2. Sleep Apnea
Syndromes—physiopathology. 3. Cardiovascular Diseases—etiology. 4.
Cardiovascular Physiological Phenomena. WF 143 L765 2010]
  RC737.5.L57 2010
  616.2—dc22

                                                    2009042891

Lippincott's Focus on Cardiovascular Disease and Sleep Apnea

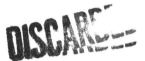

Wolters Kluwer | Lippincott Williams & Wilkins
Health
Philadelphia · Baltimore · New York · London
Buenos Aires · Hong Kong · Sydney · Tokyo

Lippincott's focus on
 cardiovascular disease and

Lippincott's Focus on Cardiovascular Disease and Sleep Apnea is adapted from

Handbook of Sleep Medicine. Avidan AY, Zee PC (eds). Lippincott Williams & Wilkins, Philadelphia. 2006

APT—Fundamentals of Sleep Technology. Butkov N and Lee-Chiong T (eds). Lippincott Williams & Wilkins, Philadelphia. 2007

Clinical Sleep Disorders. Carney PR, Berry RB, Geyer JD, (eds). Lippincott Williams & Wilkins, Philadelphia. 2005

With permission.

Adapted by Anne Scheck

CONTENTS

CHAPTER 1

Sleep Disturbances

"**A**m I going to have a heart attack if I snore?"

This is an increasingly common question from patients. Larger numbers of them who are aware they have loud breathing or engage in outright snoring during sleep are wary of that now, thanks in part to the popular press, which has reported in the last few years on the link between sleep disturbances, particularly snoring, and cardiovascular disease.

Of all the dyssomnias, disturbances that disrupt slumber, snoring is by far the most common. In the United Sates, approximately 24% of women and 40% of men habitually snore, according to findings of the Wisconsin Sleep Cohort Study. Other investigations, from Australia and Great Britain, put the number of snorers several percentage points higher among middle-aged people in those countries. Moreover, those percentages double in elderly populations in both Europe and America.

Snoring and Sleep Apnea

Snoring was once thought to be a possible precursor to sleep apnea, though not predictive of it. Now more medical literature is calling the presence of snoring a potential marker for sleep apnea, the state when air flow into lungs is fully or partly blocked and when oxygen drops to relatively dangerous levels, triggering tightening of the upper-airway muscles. The result, a characteristic

1

snort, awakens some sleepers. When this pattern persists, excessive daytime drowsiness can result.

Not all reports of such disruptions are sleep apnea, however. Upper Airway Resistance Syndrome (UARS) can be the cause: UARS is characterized by the same airway resistance and a reduction in airflow, but it does not satisfy the criteria for apnea due to the fact that stoppage is absent, too infrequent, or too short-lived to result in serious hypopnea.

Severity of hypopnea can be assessed by means of the apnea-hypopnea index (AHI):

5 to 15 Mild
15 to 50 Moderate
>50 Severe

A diagnosis of obstructive sleep apnea (OSA) should not be based on AHI alone, however. The degree of hypoxemia, the presence of irregular heart beat, the number of awakenings are all important information in assessing OSA severity.

Diagnosing Sleep Apnea

Any long-term sleep disturbance, whether apneic or UARS, is important to detect because, practically speaking, UARS, snoring and apnea all point to either partial obstruction of the airway or complete blockage of it, a growing health concern. In addition, some studies show an overwhelming majority of internet-using patients turn to online sources for self-diagnosis, and an even larger majority report using complementary or alternative medicine (CAM) to treat the self-diagnosed conditions. The Gerontological Society of America, for example, has funded polls which show that more than 85% of people 52 years of age and older have used some form of CAM—a percentage shoots to above 90% for the "very old," those 85 years and older.

Methods such as nasal strips, mouth sprays and other noninvasive approaches can be purchased over the web. Other remedies, such as tucking a sock-enclosed tennis ball into the back of a pajama top or stacking pillows three or four high into a head rest, are suggested as approaches in some of the health advice available at the touch of a few computer keystrokes.

However, snoring can be a crucial warning sign, and, at the very least, signals a problem of the air movement from the surrounding environment to and from the lungs, which occurs along a pressure gradient. The respiratory system and its mechanics are designed to produce the pressure gradients needed for breathing. When there is disruption to this system, the health cost on the individual system—the snoring person—can be high, resulting in lack of restful sleep, fatigue, low responsiveness during daytime activities, reduced motor skills and even depression.

Snoring: The Impact on Bed Partners

Of all the disturbances of sleep, only snoring involves complaints from two different patient groups: the sufferers themselves, who are often awakened by their own noisy slumber, and their spouses, bed partners or family members who have the same reaction. In some ways this is advantageous—snoring is an indication of potential sleep apnea, and often spouses are responsible for ensuring it is brought to medical attention.

About one-third of the elderly report poor sleep or sleep difficulties and many of these troubled sleepers are kept from slumber by snoring bed partners. Awakenings by a partner's snoring can number close to two dozen in a single night, according to a study by investigators at the Mayo Clinic in Rochester, MN. Additionally, these bed partners are at about the same risk of daytime drowsiness as their partners who wake from apneic episodes. The situation also takes an emotional toll.

When the *New York Times* reported on snoring as a special feature article in the summer of 2009, there were anecdotal reports—some in the form of direct responses to the article after it appeared—that snoring puts a strain on marriage. One respondent compared her sleeping husband to a "lawn mower," noting that she had to kick him "harder than Beckham with a soccer ball" to get through the night, and concluded: "We both slept much better when single."

The arousals can lead to insomnia, or at least brief periods of it, on the part of both bed partners, a situation that can cause cardiovascular risk to both. Insomnia and sleep apnea both are associated with increased risk of cardiovascular disease. Some studies indicate, in fact, that insomnia predicts a slight, but measurable, increased risk of cardiovascular disease (1).

Sleep Disruption: Morbidity and Mortality

Sleep-disordered breathing is commonly associated with adverse health outcomes, such as hypertension, stroke and cardiovascular disease. Hypopneas that show desaturation of at least 4%, for example, are associated with cardiovascular disease (2). In a study of more than 6,000 adults, those who had night-time arousals consistent with sleep-disordered breathing were evaluated on the basis of AHI; hypopnea measures that showed less than 4% hemoglobin desaturation or presence of arousals showed no association with cardiovascular disease. However, an independent association was found when the level reached 4% or higher. This investigation followed another in which cyclic intermittent hypoxia was created for a group of 18 healthy volunteers, by having them sleep in a hypoxic tent to artificially impose repetitive cycles of desaturation and reoxygenation (3). The aim was to determine the plausibility of a pathogenic link in ordinary human participants. Waking normoxic arterial pressure increased significantly, supporting the link—and providing a possible way to study it.

Mortality also has been similarly documented by some of the same investigators that have demonstrated the association with morbidity. In a large multi-center study, the Sleep heart Health Study, sleep-disordered breathing was found to be associated with an increased risk of death from any cause in nearly 6,300 men and women who participated in it. The study, funded by the National Heart, Lung and Blood Institute, included 10 institutions (4).

Sleep disordered breathing was assessed with the AHI. The average follow-up period was more than eight years. Sleep-related intermittent hypoxemia was independently related to all-cause mortality; coronary artery disease-related mortality associated with sleep-disordered breathing showed a pattern of association similar to all-cause mortality.

Obstructive Sleep Apnea

Sleep apnea can be found in more than half of patients older than 70. OSA, caused by an airway obstruction, is more common; central sleep apnea, caused by a disruption in signaling that ordinarily stimulates and assures normal respiration, is less common. Because the two so often occur concurrently, they often are referred to under the common term "sleep apnea."

Obesity, as measured by a BMI >30 kg per m², and advancing age (>65 years), are primary risk factors for OSA. The relationship between OSA and ischemic heart disease, arrhythmias, stroke and coronary artery disease have been examined, and risk well established in the number of motor vehicle accidents related to daytime sleepiness.

OSA evaluation combines historical data, physical examination, and nocturnal polysomnography to determine the presence of daytime symptoms, apnea or hypopnea, hypoxemia, arousals, respiratory effort, and any disturbances in sleep architecture.

Symptoms of OSA

- Daytime sleepiness
- Chronic fatigue
- Morning headaches
- Restless sleep
- Insomnia
- Depression
- Sexual problems
- Nasal congestion

The Assessment of Sleep Apnea by Polysomnography

There are no definite recommendations for when such sleep-lab studies should be performed. Obesity and snoring both are linked to OSA, and both to cardiovascular risk factors. As obesity rates rocket, a debate has arisen as to the clinical necessity for more polysomnography. The situation has been perplexing: Obesity is usually defined by Body Mass Index (BMI) but BMI provides scant indication of the location of body fat. However, obese people sometimes are surprisingly free of obvious health complications, and so are individuals who report—or are reported to have—heavy snoring.

Question-and-answer tools, such as the Berlin Questionnaire, can help identify such patients by asking straightforward inquiries such as "Do you snore?" and "Has your snoring bothered other people?"

A scoring rubric is used to determine if the answers are cause for further investigation. Other, similar surveys, such as Canada's Public Health sleep inventory form and the Stanford Scale (Table 1.1) also can help pinpoint problem sleepers. Because sleep apnea can have substantial impact on emotional well-being, as well as cardiovascular risk, there is increasing support for wider use of polysomnography. In the past, such sleep studies were often reserved for those with frank symptoms.

By using electroencephalography (ECG), along with the Epworth test—a sleepiness scale in which likelihood of dozing is determined—researchers were able to more accurately confirm suspicion of OSA.

Holter monitoring, overnight oximetry and even respiratory distress indices all were suggested as alternate screening tests. Sleep diaries and other self-report measures are still relied upon, but frequently, are followed by polysomnography (PSG).

However, without polysomnography, distinction of pathology is challenging: The main controversy with other screening approaches, including sensitive devices that monitor pressure swings such as nasal cannula-pressure transducers, is that subtle decreases in air flow are not as easily detected. With ECG, some patients only exhibit irregular rhythms during sleep,

Table 1.1	Stanford Sleepiness Scale	
Degrees of Sleepiness		Scale Rating
Feeling active, vital, alert, or wide awake		1
Functioning at high levels, but not at peak; able to concentrate		2
Awake, but relaxed; responsive but not fully alert		3
Somewhat foggy, let down		4
Foggy; losing interest in remaining awake; slowed down		5
Sleepy, woozy, fighting sleep; prefer to lie down		6
No longer fighting sleep, sleep onset soon; having dream-like thoughts		7
Asleep		X

Accompanying text to Stanford Sleepiness Scale:

This is a quick way to assess how alert you are feeling. If it is during the day when you go about your business, ideally you would want a rating of a one. Take into account that most people have two peak times of alertness daily, at about 9 a.m. and 9 p.m. Alertness wanes to its lowest point at around 3 p.m.; after that it begins to build again. Rate your alertness at different times during the day. If you go below a three when you should be feeling alert, this is an indication that you have a serious sleep debt and you need more sleep.

especially if they suffer from sleep-disordered breathing, while having a more normal rate and rhythm during waking hours.

Nocturnal Polysomnography

Nocturnal PSG is a procedure carried out in a sleep laboratory, and it involves extensive monitoring. When the decision is made to evaluate a patient by this means, the laboratory typically needs 2–3 hours to prepare for the test before bedtime.

Polysomnograms are both more sensitive and more specific—enabling the diagnosis of OSA and its severity. The quality of the polygraphs depends on the techniques employed.

Obstructive apnea or hypoapnea is noted on the polygraph when airflow is reduced or absent, but obvious chest or abdominal motion is detected as well, indicating an attempt by the patient to breath. Hypoxemia is demonstrated by a reduction in SpO_2—(oxygen saturation as measured by pulse oximetry)—during episodes of apnea or hypopnea.

Apnea during sleep can result from an obstruction of the upper pharynx and/or loss of ventilatory effort. The latter condition, know as *central sleep apnea*, is characterized by frequent episodes of decreased airflow in the absence of respiratory effort. OSA is associated with obvious ventilatory effort that occurs during apnea or hypopnea.

Polysomnography can distinguish between the two. OSA is by far more prevalent and the typical reason that sleep studies are undertaken.

The incidence of snoring occurs in all stages of sleep but primarily the second and fourth, the stages which constitute the longest and deepest respectively.

Men are more likely to have sleep apnea than premenopausal women; however, the incidence in women increases after menopause. These influences can also be impacted by ethnicity. African Americans, Asians, and Hispanics seem to be at an increased risk for severe apnea, though it has yet to be determined why.

Snoring, once thought to be a possible precursor but not predictive of sleep apnea, is proving to be a marker for it, but only when the snoring is persistent, associated with sleep that is not particularly restful and linked to excessive day time sleepiness, and when the patient has reported night-time awakenings from what has been called a "resuscitative snort."

However, snoring can be a warning sign of apnea. Practically speaking, snoring is partial obstruction of the airway, apnea is complete blockage of it. For a majority of Americans entering their sixth decade, it can be a danger signal—OSA.

References

1. Phillips B, Mannino D. Do insomnia complaints cause hypertension or cardiovascular disease? *J Clin Sleep Med* 3(5):89–94, 2007.
2. Punjabi N, Newman A, Young T, et al. American Sleep-disordered breathing and cardiovascular disease: an outcome-based definition of hypopneas. *J Respiratory and Critical Care Medicine* 177:1150–1155, 2008.
3. Tamisier R, Gilmartin G, Launois S, et al. A new model of chronic intermittent hypoxia in humans: effect on ventilation, sleep, and blood pressure. *J Appl Physiol* 107(1):17–24, 2009.
4. Punjabi N, Caffo B, Goodwin J, et al. Sleep-disordered breathing and mortality: a prospective cohort study. *PLoS Med* 6(8), 2009.

CHAPTER **2**

Obstructive Sleep Apnea

The prevalence of obstructive sleep apnea (OSA) is increasing as two risk factors for it, obesity and old age, become far more common. The baby boom cohort continues to swell the retirement-age population and obesity is now at epidemic proportions. As a result, OSA is estimated to have doubled among the general population—to nearly one in 10 adults—up from about 5% only a decade ago. As patient groups that are overweight or past 65 years of age continue to grow, so does the likelihood of OSA. In the near future, in fact, the doubling will occur much sooner, possibly in the next five years.

Every eight seconds, another American is reaching the traditional retirement age, adding yet another potentially OSA-susceptible candidate to the population. Currently, the 85-and-older group is now rising faster than any other, and that trend is expected to continue in the near future (1). It is also worth noting that this group of newly elderly people differs from the preceding one—the boom generation has proven itself to be more demanding of medical care, and unlikely to accept more restrained activities of daily living later in life, compared with its predecessor. More older adults than ever before want to continue living independently, with as high a quality of life as possible provided through medical intervention (2).

An Overview of OSA

The classic definition of OSA is complete collapse of the airway, leading to a stoppage in breathing of 10 seconds or more, although many patients have apnea far exceeding the 10-second cut-off. To assess OSA severity, the apnea-hypoxia index often is used, a ratio that compares the number apneic and hypopneic periods during one hour. Most normal sleepers have less than five; Most OSA patients have more than five, and many have more than 10.

OSA seems gender-related, if not gender-specific. In elderly men, the rate of OSA has been found to be as high as 40%, compared with a 3% to 6% incidence in women of comparable age. However, research has shown that the condition often goes undiagnosed in both sexes, even though symptoms may be persistent. Such signs include daytime drowsiness, general fatigue, clumsiness in performing routine tasks, problems in concentration, and subtle impairments of memory and judgment. Personality changes also may occur, especially heightened irritability and anxiety. But because memory lapses, lower energy and even personality differences often are associated with the aging process itself, the potential underlying cause of OSA may be overlooked.

In fact, one of the most frequent ways in which OSA comes to medical attention is by way of a spouse, partner or family member who expresses concern over a pattern of snoring and breathlessness by a loved one during sleep. Often, this worry arises when snoring stops for a time, usually 20 to 30 seconds of breathing cessation, that is followed by a loud gasp or snort. A spouse or partner may report this episode as frightening—a period in which they feared the sleeping person would not wake up or that the gasping meant there was difficulty in resuming normal breathing. These experiences also may awaken the sleeping person, but he or she may attribute such awakenings to insomnia.

Because insomnia is a relatively common complaint, and because there are now effective medications to curb it, OSA-associated insomnia episodes may escape early diagnosis—but

OSA poses a health risk as soon as it begins, due to its association with other morbidity, particularly those of cardiovascular disease.

Conditions Associated with Sleep Apnea

Hypertension

Studies suggest a strong, direct relationship between systemic hypertension and OSA. OSA occurs in about a third of hypertensive patients and half or more of all patients diagnosed with OSA also are hypertensive. In addition, hypertensive patients who have OSA show significantly higher blood pressure and heart rates, even during sleep, compared to age-matched counterparts in control groups who don't experience sleep apnea. As a result, OSA is considered a risk factor for hypertension, and hypertensive patients are considered at risk for OSA.

How does this relationship exist? Apparently, from sympathetic over-activity initiated by hypoxemia, which causes sleep interruptions. In turn, the fluctuations in blood pressure during these periodic arousals play a role in hypertension. Compelling evidence that this chain of events may constitute a cause-and-effect relationship comes from research that demonstrates hypertension can be reduced or reversed once OSA is successfully treated.

Heart Disease

Many studies, including several investigations by the American Heart Association, have linked both ischemia and arrhythmia to OSA. Some of the findings show strong associations between oscillations in pulmonary artery pressure, sleep apneas and nocturnal angina in patients with OSA and a history of heart disease. In one prospective study, for example, patients with OSA were found to have much higher numbers—and levels—of serologic markers for risk for cardiac disease, such as leptin, C-reactive protein and homocystine.

Cerebrovascular Disease

Because OSA and hypertension are often concomitant, OSA may put patients who have not been diagnosed with either condition at risk for cerebrovascular events, such as stroke. This increased risk can be explained etiologically on the basis of impairments in endothelial function, which predispose atherogenesis and, without intervention, can lead to thrombosis and embolism. In one study of more than 100 late-middle-aged men who both snored and reported disturbances in night-time slumber, there was significantly greater thickening of carotid arteries and more presence of plaque, compared with men who snored but did not have such sleep interruptions.

Prevalence of sleep-disordered breathing in acute stroke patients ranges between 44% and 95% compared with prevalence in the community to between 9% and 35% in women and 8% and 57% in men (3, 4).

Quality of Life Issues

For people with OSA, the interruptions in sleep may not be noticeable. For their bed partners, they may become an accepted part of the sleep cycle. But learning to live with OSA can have serious consequences on quality of life, as well as general health. Activities of daily living may be severely affected, including driving against waves of drowsiness or struggling to maintain attentiveness.

Loss of focus and retention during conversations and flares of temper over incidents that others may consider trivial can inflict injury on personal and family support. All of this can become a frustrating situation, and not just for the person with OSA but for the people around him or her, who may become anxious and overwhelmed around a person they have known and loved. If OSA goes undiagnosed, such symptoms not only persist, but may progress—ending in an outcome that may leave an OSA sufferer in far worse shape, as health deteriorates and family members become less understanding.

Diagnosis

Physical Examination

OSA should be suspected in patients who have a body mass index indicative of obesity or a neck circumference of greater than 40 centimeters, particularly when they are found in patients more than 40 years of age. For patients 65 years of age or more who meet such criteria, OSA should be considered presumptively until testing proves otherwise. The most common test is by means of an apnea-hypoxia index.

Initially, oral and nasal cavities need to be assessed in these patients. Septal asymmetry or enlarged turbinates in nasal passages should raise the index of suspicion. A simple clinical test for the oral cavity is the Mallampatti scale, in which a patient is requested to open his or her mouth as wide as possible and to stick out the tongue. In this way, the soft palate, the uvula, the lateral pillars, and the tongue can be examined. Bulging or "kissing" tonsils, an abnormal-looking uvula, and the presence of a bony structure, such as a narrow or high arched palate, are all morphological characteristics associated with OSA.

In the Mallampatti scale, the degree of pharyngeal crowding is scored from "one to four." "One" designates an unobstructed, wide orophyarynx in which the uvula is clearly above the tongue; "Two" designates visibility of the pillars and at least part of the inferior segment of the uvula. "Three" reflects a substantially more limited visualization of the oropharynx—a barely visible uvula, for example. "Four" shows a crowded oropharynx with only the hard palate visible (the uvula is obscured by the tongue). Scores of "three" or "four" have been associated with difficulty in breathing, which may be tolerated by the patient during waking hours but are exacerbated during sleep. These scores should be considered a sign for investigation of possible OSA.

Patient History

A history of snoring can be an important indicator of OSA, though it is not definitive—snoring by itself is not an established risk factor for OSA. However, a majority of patients who snore and complain of daytime drowsiness have been found to have OSA after further diagnostic testing. Though insomnia is another possible marker for OSA, it alone is unreliable. Neither sleepwalking nor sleeplessness is indicative of OSA. It is the periodic awakenings without explanation that are attributed to insomnia that point to OSA as a possible etiology. Patients with OSA are more likely to complain of daytime fatigue and nonspecific somatic complaints.

A specific type of OSA as defined by the American Academy of Sleep Medicine Task Force is upper-airway resistance syndrome (URAS). General symptoms of URAS match those of OSA, although about half of URAS patients experience cold hands and feet and about a third feel light-headed when they stand quickly. Some researchers believe the two syndromes—URAS and OSA—should be considered distinct, clinical entities.

Diagnostic Tests

Full-night Polysomnography

For patients who are suspected of having URAS or OSA, polysomnography is routinely recommended, and most often the studies are done at a sleep lab. Usually, this consists of continual monitoring during sleep by electroencephalogram; Electro-oculograms and recordings of muscle activity of the upper body also often are taken. Arterial oxyhemoglobin saturation studies may be included, as well as urinary catecholamine measures. In general, 24-hour electrocardiagrams are done for patients in whom heart disease is suspected or has been diagnosed.

The esophageal-pressure monitoring that is done during polysomnography can record even subtle changes in respiration, pulse and arterial flow. Are there increases in inspiratory falls of blood pressure? Other alterations of blood pressure during times of sleep arousal? Polysomnography detects such differences. Adults with OSA generally experience five OSA incidents during every hour of sleep, and each lasts at least ten seconds. Often, confirmation of OSA is made on the basis of these frequent sleep arousals when arterial oxygen desaturation or bradytachycardia also occurs.

Split-night Polysomnography

Split-night polysomnography involves diagnostic recordings, in conjunction with the use of continuous of positive airway pressure (CPAP) titration. The aim of this split-time approach is to establish a baseline during the first half of sleep, and then to determine if symptoms are diminished with the use of CPAP during the second half. Traditionally, split-night polysomnography refers to diagnostic recordings followed by CPAP during the same night. However, sometimes a full night of polysomnography may be warranted, followed by a full night of CPAP. Alternatively, a split-night polysomnography may be done, with diagnostic testing followed by CPAP. In fact, a second night of CPAP may be undertaken. Second-night CPAP offers a broader picture of symptom control, and can give a clearer indication of whether the treatment is effective.

References

1. Jurkowski E. Policy and program planning for older adults: realities and visions. Springer Publishing Company, New York, 2008.
2. Kane R. Coalitions between aging and disability interests: a potential vehicle to promote community care for older people. In Putnam M., editor: Aging and disability: Crossing network lines. Springer Publishing Company, New York, 2007.
3. Cadihac D, Thorpe R, Pearce D, et al. SCOPES II Study Group. Sleep disordered breathing in congestive stroke survivors. A study of the long term follow-up of the SCOPES cohort using home based polysomnography. *J Clin Neurosci* 2005;12:632–637.
4. Parra O, Arboix A, Montserrat J, et al. Sleep-related breathing disorders: impact on mortality of cerebrovascular disease. *Eur Respir J* 2004;24:267–272.

CHAPTER 3

Central Sleep Apnea

Central sleep apnea (CSA) is a syndrome in which repeated interruptions in breathing occur during sleep due to loss of ventilatory effort. It is distinguished from obstructive sleep apnea (OSA) because sleep disturbances do not arise from upper airway obstruction but rather, from lapses in ventilation. However, many patients with OSA have CSA and vice versa, making this overlap of syndromes typical—and the lack of such overlap unusual. In fact, patients who predominantly have CSA number fewer than one in ten patients in most sleep-lab studies and some estimates have put these patients at less than 5% of the entire population with sleep apnea.

However, there is anecdotal evidence that CSA may be seriously under-recognized, at least until it coexists with OSA. Many cases of sleep apnea are detected either by a gasping snorer who awakens to resume breathing after a sensation of suffocation or by a bed partner who is awakened when that happens. The lack of respiratory effort that ensues during CSA often results in no such openly dramatic fights for breath—and the person who has CSA may be unaware of the night-time breathing difficulty, even when the irregular breathing causes an awakening. Unlike OSA, complete cessation due to blockage of breathing is unlikely to occur. Rather, there is crescendo-decrescendo pattern of tidal volume in which the partial pressure of CO_2 drops so far that the apnea results.

CSA most commonly is linked to congestive heart failure (CHF), an association so strong that CSA is a marker for heart disease and patients who are diagnosed with CHF are presumed to have CSA as an underlying cause of sleep-related difficulty.

The absence of the central respiratory drive to function normally in CSA likely stems from chemical imbalances in the brain, although the precise etiology still remains largely unexplained in the absence of obvious causes, such as drug use or a comorbid condition. What is known is that the respiration system does not seem to respond effectively to the delicate feedback mechanisms involving carbon dioxide. As a result, CSA characteristically becomes a state in which apnea alternates with hyperpnea.

The periodic loss of ventilatory control in CSA, though not characterized by stoppage from obstruction, nonetheless renders breathing a series of fits and starts during slumber—the result most often of hypoventilation. This hypoventilation may arise in the presence of a heritable or chronic condition, such as Ondine's Curse, in which breathing results in hypercapnia and hypoxemia, or more commonly, Pickwickian Syndrome, in which obesity-related sleep apnea occurs. Other causes of this hypoventilation include the use of narcotic medications, age-related changes in the processes involved in the transition from wakefulness to sleep and abnormalities in the respiratory control system due to injury or disease, such as chest trauma or lung infection. Though rare, cases of CSA in which no etiology can be found do occur, and they fall into a distinct category: idiopathic CSA.

In many individuals with CHF, breathing not only fluctuates during sleep—waxing, waning, stopping and starting—but the pattern is marked by a relatively prolonged ventilatory phase, even when compared with other patients who have sleep apneas. When the ventilation pattern in these heart patients alternates between rapid breathing and extreme slowing or cessation of breath, Cheyne-Stokes respiration is occurring. In fact, some investigators use Cheyne-Stokes interchangeably with CSA, as the two are so commonly linked. Cheyne-Stokes, typically, signals that both CHF and CSA are occurring, even in the absence of other physical indications.

Cheyne-Stokes Respiration

The most obvious presentation of Cheyne-Stokes is a pattern of recurrent respiration in which there is fast breath-taking—either deep or shallow—followed by apnea. The syndrome also is seen in patients who have neurologic conditions, particularly those with cerebrovascular complications, such as stroke sequelae. On clinical measures, patients with Cheyne-Stokes respiration, typically have lower levels of pCO_2 during wakefulness than do CHF patients who do not have Cheyne-Stokes respiration. They also have relatively low arterial oxygen saturation during sleep.

The specific reason underlying these abnormal blood gases in Cheyne-Stokes respiration has not been determined, but the association between CHF and Cheyne-Stokes respiration suggests that cardiac dysfunction may play a significant role, influencing ventilation in a way that inhibits or destabilizes it—though the major underlying mechanism causing fluctuations in the serum partial pressures of carbon dioxide remains unknown. There is evidence of heightened chemosensitivity to hypoxia and hypercapnia in CHF patients during late-stage disease. In fact, the combination of enhanced chemosensitivity to both low oxygen and high carbon dioxide has been suggested to have prognostic value for patients with heart failure (1).

Hypercapnia and Hypocapnia in CSA

Some patients with CSA appear to have defective pathways driving ventilation—chemoreceptor anomalies or deficiencies that seem to relate only to abnormally high or low sensitivity to pCO_2, pO_2 or hydrogen. In addition, some studies suggest there are as-yet unknown barriers to translation of essential chemical information to ventilatory drives—the pathophysiological equivalent of errant cross-wiring. Another possibility is that certain subtle anatomical differences affect the performance in ways that have yet to be qualified. Regardless of the specific underlying reason, when such abnormalities cause under-ventilation, they result in a form of CSA known *hypercapnia*, which causes higher-than-normal levels of carbon dioxide to accumulate in blood. When such abnormalities cause over-ventilation, they cause a form of CSA known as *hypocapnia*. Most CSA patients are hypercapnic, and of those, the most severe episodes of hypoventilation largely occur during the REM stages of sleep, a physiologically distinct phase of slumber where dreams occur and sometimes register in memory. As a result, night-time arousal related to CSA may be attributed to awakenings from vivid mental scenarios. Unfortunately, in the absence of a polysomnogram, these patients can be difficult to identify without obvious symptoms of the sleep-disorder breathing.

Reasons to suspect hypercapnia CSA include an elevated bicarbonate level, evidence of peripheral edema or right-heart failure, and major hypoxemia and hypercapnia during respiratory infection. Complaints of fatigue and weakness among these patients constitute another clinical sign, as does positional dyspnea or orthopnea in the presence of diaphragm weakness. In the case of diaphragm weakness, physical examination may reveal respiratory paradox during a supine body position. Arterial blood gas studies on patients with normal lung parenchyma also can help identify hypercapnia, which typically causes chronic respiratory acidosis in these patients. An elevated pCO_2, with a low normal pH and a preserved $A\text{-}aDO_2$ gradients, also raise the index of suspicion that hypoventilation is occurring. Evaluations by the Sniff Test, esophageal balloon study or diaphragm ultrasound can help identify such patients, as well, though these tests probably are best reserved for more questionable presentations. Measurement of respiratory muscle pressure—maximal inspiratory pressure plus maximal expiratory pressure—also can be used, though this method assesses the neuromuscular reflexivity and is not diagnostic for hypercapnia. Spirometry is another helpful tool: If a substantial decline in vital capacity is observed between the upright and supine posture, hypercapnia may be presumed.

Hypercapnic CSA and Hypoventilation Syndrome

Although patients with hypercapnia may appear to breathe normally the daytime, they usually also have hypercapnia during the day, which worsens with sleep at night. And, because some of these patients fail to show multiple CSA episodes during sleep studies, they are put in a special category by some researchers known as "hypoventilation syndrome," which has been attributed to defects in central drive but not in the motor nerves, spinal cord, respiratory muscles or lungs. Injury to the chest wall and lungs also can lead to this syndrome, as can many autoimmune diseases, such as amyotrophic lateral sclerosis.

Therefore, patients with lung or chest abnormalities—or any disorder affecting ventilatory control—may respond to treatment, as studies with CPAP in these patients have shown. In general, mechanical ventilation is the treatment of choice for hypercapnia in which no frank abnormalities can be found. For such patients, nasal or nasal-oral masks and a pressure-cycled or volume-cycled ventilator can restore nocturnal ventilation. Nasal bi-level positive airway pressure has become a standard treatment for hypercapnic CSA.

Non-hypercapnic CSA

Non-hypercapnic forms of CSA are said to represent a distinct clinical presentation because the $paCO_2$ levels are normal or low, in contrast to hypercapnic CSA, in which they are often found to be elevated (2).

The most common form of non-hypercapnic syndrome is Cheyne-Stokes respiration. Because it has become a marker for potentially poor cardiac function, treatment of non-hypercapnic syndrome with Cheyne-Stokes is critical. CPAP seems to lower the resistance in the upper airway, however, which leads to falls in pCO_2. A similar phenomenon seems to occur following tracheostomy. In both treatment approaches, these apnea incidents often are found to resolve with time.

CSA, OSA and Quality of Life

Both OSA and CSA are common in heart failure, and most individuals with both disorders either have congestive heart failure or progress to it. The impact of this sleep disordered breathing has an effect detrimental to quality of life before such progression, however, and if detected and with treatment, quality of life can be preserved (3). Can early detection of CSA, OSA or both prevent the onset of cardiac disease and related cardiovascular complications, such as atherosclerosis and high blood pressure? There is a growing body of evidence that suggests just that, as the link between heart disease and sleep apnea is explored more intensely in research designed to establish the pathology that underlies the sleep disruptions that grow more common with age, weight gain and some comorbid conditions.

References

1. Giannoni A, Emdin M, Bramanti F, et al. Combined increased chemosensitivity to hypoxia and hypercapnia as a prognosticator in heart failure. *J Am College of Cardiology* 53(21):1975–1980, 2009.
2. Yumino D, Bradley T. Central sleep apnea and Cheyne-Stokes respiration. *Proc Am Thorac Soc.* 5(2):226–236, 2008.
3. Skobel E, Norra C, Sinha A, et al. Sleep and quality of life in heart failure and stroke. In Verester J, Pandi-Perumal S, Streiner D (eds). Sleep and quality of life in clinical medicine. Humana Press, Totowa, NJ, 2008.

CHAPTER 4

Obstructive Sleep Apnea and Heart Disease

Changes in blood flow occur with obstructive sleep apnea (OSA), increasing both cardiovascular risk, progression to more severe disease for those in the early stages of it, and the development of hypertension in patients prone to high blood pressure. How does this happen? In untreated OSA, peripheral blood flow undergoes vasoconstriction and there is intermittent hypoxemia and CO_2 retention. Thus, OSA doesn't just disturb the quality of slumber, it causes oxygenation to plunge, to ≤60% at times. And, toward the end of such episodes, blood pressure may climb to 240/130 mmHg—a level of hemodynamic stress that can contribute to encroaching heart disease. Even healthy people with OSA have higher heart rates during periods of wakefulness compared with others who do not experience OSA. The reason for this, theoretically, is that there is an increased sympathetic drive that persists even during normal daytime activities. Evidence for that can be found in studies of patients with OSA, many of whom show this heart-rate escalation. Moreover, when given 100% oxygen to lower the responses that heighten sympathetic activity, both heart rate and blood pressure go down in patients with OSA during wakeful periods.

The ways in which untreated OSA may heighten cardiovascular risk were gleaned from extant research and published in 2008 as "Sleep Apnea and Cardiovascular Disease," a joint scientific statement by American Heart Association and the American College of Cardiology Foundation. A summary of findings from the publication:

1. **OSA is associated with less cardiovascular variability.** OSA patients have less heart-rate variability and more blood pressure variability, compared with people who have no OSA. Lower heart-rate variability not only is a known risk factor for cardiovascular disease, evidence of it is a marker for a potentially poor outcome. This high-variability pattern also is associated with the development of hypertension, and in turn, with increased end-stage organ damage.

2. **OSA appears to initiate inflammation.** The sleep disruption caused by OSA appears to trigger inflammation in two ways: specifically, the recurrent hypoxemia activates pro-inflammatory transcription factor (nuclear factor K-B); and, more generally, there is selective activation of inflammatory pathways—rather than adaptive ones.

3. **Hypoxemic stress linked to OSA increases vasoconstriction.** Hypoxia is associated with induction that increases the release of vasoactive and trophic substances, constricting vessels. Sleep apnea that is untreated also raises endothelin levels, a finding that may help explain the theoretical link to endothelial dysfunction in OSA. Results of some studies suggest a cause-and-effect relationship between stress, increased endothelin production and endothelial dysfunction, though the findings are not universally consistent.

4. **Insulin resistance rises when OSA occurs.** Some research has found an association between glucose intolerance and OSA, apart from diabetes or body-mass index measures. Leptin resistance also has been documented in patient groups with OSA.

5. **OSA leads to intrathoracic pressure changes that alter ventricular function.** Impaired diastolic function can result from the negative pressure to the chest cavity caused by repeated, forceful inspiration against the closed upper airway; Other potential consequences of this abnormal respiration are

thoracic aortic dilation, propensity toward dissection, increased wall stress and increased atrial size.

Under persistent and untreated OSA, these nocturnal episodes may lead to ventricular remodeling. Untreated OSA has been shown to disrupt ventricular function and autonomic and hemodynamic stability—and not just temporarily. Though such a causative link has yet to be firmly established, the resulting negative intrathoracic pressure has been shown to increase transmural gradients across the ventricles, aorta and the atria, presumably setting the stage for ventricular change, including hypertrophy.

6. **Severe OSA has been implicated in blood-flow impairment.** Increased platelet activation and increased fibrinogen both have been associated with recurrent OSA. In addition, there is an inverse relationship between brachial artery-mediated flow and sleep-apnea severity in patients with co-morbidities.

7. **OSA may trigger oxidative-stress mechanisms.** Studies comparing measures of gene transcription in OSA patients during sleep and wakeful times suggest overnight hypoxemia triggers controlling signals for oxidative stress mechanisms. Some investigations have found increases in oxidized low-density lipoprotein in OSA, but such an association has not been confirmed in other studies.

The possible role of OSA in hypertension has been elucidated in animal studies, as well, which show that there is increased sensitivity in the renin-angiotensin system. When OSA is artificially created in dogs, for example, there is a marked triggering of the sympathetic response—just as is seen in human studies on cardiovascular disease. Studies on both hypertension and cardiovascular disease generally point to the apparent impact of hypoxemic stress of OSA.

OSA has been so strongly implicated in hypertension, in fact, that it increasingly is seen as an independent risk factor for essential hypertension. In the Wisconsin Sleep Cohort Study, for example, a consistent dose-response relationship was established between OSA and blood pressure, even after investigators controlled for age, gender, body-mass index and anti-hypertensive medications. In addition, treatment with continuous positive airway pressure has been shown to dramatically reduce blood pressure in hypertensive patients during sleep. OSA has also been identified as an important, identifiable cause of hypertension by several research groups.

OSA Severity as a Marker for Heart Disease

Patients with OSA have a high prevalence of coronary artery disease and there is a high incidence of OSA in patients with CHF, as well. As a result, OSA can be considered an independent risk factor for heart disease, as well as for hypertension. What accounts for the risk? When polysomnograms of snorers who have apnea have been compared with those who don't experience OSA, the snoring patients with this form of apnea have been found to have more frequent incidents of ST segment depression, sinus bradycardia and sinus pauses; conversely, when polysomnograms are conducted on healthy volunteers, such potentially pathologic breathing changes, as measured by respiratory disruptive events per hour of sleep, don't usually occur in patients who are younger and in good health, but dramatically increase in patients older than 50 (1).

Other research has shown that, when such episodes lead to hypercapnia, there is apparent activation of the sympathetic nervous system. However, establishing a definitive causative relationship, rather than an association, between sleep apnea and cardiovascular disease has been elusive. Recent studies help explain how it may happen, however.

There is some evidence that OSA actually initiates cardiac ischemia. In one study of more than 200 consecutive patients without a history of coronary artery disease who had undergone polysomnography within the past three years, arterial calicifications scores were relatively high in the OSA patients and non-existent in a control group without OSA. In addition, the calcification scores increased along with worsening OSA severity. The results of the calcification measures appear to confirm an independent association between OSA and subclinical coronary artery disease, the authors concluded (2).

Moreover, studies on patients with myocardial ischemia demonstrate two associations of clinical importance: that untreated OSA is associated with more cardiovascular events, both fatal and non-fatal and additionally, that treatment seems to confer protection against such events. In fact, cardiovascular events in some treatment groups approach that of traditional snorers who have no history of OSA. Also, nocturnal arrhythmias have been found to be more common in OSA patients, and their occurrence seems to be related to the severity of OSA. Studies indicate the risk can be mitigated with treatment, through use of continuous positive airway pressure (CPAP), and studies suggest this restoration of air flow can reverse some of the suspected pathologic mechanisms that may exacerbate heart disease.

Treatment with CPAP is associated with decreases in echocardiographic measures, suggesting it mitigates pulmonary hypertension. In studies of patients with elevated pulmonary pressure who have OSA, the pressures typically fall post-treatment with CPAP. The likely mechanism underlying this form of hypertension has been theorized to be hypoxemia, although proof that this process during OSA is an actual cause of pulmonary arterial hypertension is confounded by the fact that these patients also are obese, and obesity is itself considered a frequent co-factor for both OSA and pulmonary arterial hypertension.

Concurrence of Obesity, OSA and Heart Disease

Obesity is an independent risk factor for both cardiovascular disease and OSA. Currently, a majority of adult Americans are now either overweight or obese, according to the National Health and Nutrition Examination Survey—a finding that helps explains the rise in OSA and the reason that cardiovascular disease causes the most mortality in the United States. Obesity and OSA seem to share some common pathology: increases in oxidative stress, endothelial dysfunction and heightened inflammatory responses (2).

Are there shared and unshared genetic factors that underlie susceptibility to both OSA and obesity, and by inference, cardiovascular disease? Genome scans in a series of Caucasian volunteers suggest there may be a common causal pathway involving regulation of both the apnea-hypopnea index and body mass index (3). Because OSA pathways may lead to atherosclerosis, hypertension and insulin resistance, some sleep researchers propose all patients with severe sleep apnea should be treated, to reduce cardiovascular risk. Weight loss has been found to at least partially reduce the incidence of OSA, so that approach is now recommended as well, to reduce the risk of morbidity and mortality. Because obesity is reaching epidemic proportions, even in young children, it is becoming an intense focus of research. Does normal weight prevent the onset of OSA, CSA and the presumed influence of such sleep disruptions on heart disease? There is evidence that it does, and that evidence is accumulating.

References

1. Pavlova M, Duffy J, Shea S. Polysomnographic respiratory abnormalities in asymptomatic individuals. *Sleep* 1;31(2):241–248, 2008.
2. Iqbal M, Shah S, Fernandez S, et al. Obesity, obstructive sleep apnea, and cardiovascular risk. *Current Cardiovascular Risk Reports* 2(2): 101–106, 2008.
3. Palmer L, Buxbaum S, Larkin E, et al. A whole-genome scan for obstructive sleep apnea and obesity. *Am J Hum Genet* 72(2):340–350, 2003.

CHAPTER 5

Comorbidities and Obstructive Sleep Apnea

A 55-year-old man arrives for his annual health check-up. He is short of breath, even though he has just walked in from a parking space only 10 yards from the medical office suite. He tries to catch his breath, pausing frequently, as he composes sentences in short bursts, blurting out of only a few words at a time. He is leaning on his "walking stick," while insisting the reason he made an appointment is just routine—except for a slight tightness in his chest, that is. But the pain comes and goes every so often, and it doesn't worry him that much. He is almost six feet tall, but stout. His records indicate a body-mass index of 59.5 kg/m^2. His ankles are swollen, but they cause him no discomfort, he says. In fact, he doesn't have anything wrong, he insists, nothing that a good night's sleep wouldn't cure, anyway.

What is a good night's sleep? A night divided into two types of continual sleep: rapid eye movement (REM) sleep and non-REM sleep. (Table 5.1.) Typically, sleep begins with light, non-REM sleep. In stage 1, sleep is *very* light, and awakening occurs frequently, often from noises or other disturbances. During this first stage of sleep, eyes move slowly, and muscle activity slows. Then stage 2 non-REM sleep commences, and eye movements stop. The brain shows a distinctive pattern of slower brain waves with occasional bursts of rapid waves. When there is progression into stage 3 non-REM sleep, the brain waves become even

Table 5.1	The Five Phases of Sleep
Stage 1	Light sleep, brain waves fairly undifferentiated
Stage 2	Light sleep, brain waves begin to slow (50% delta)
Stage 3	Deep sleep, brain waves continue slowing (more delta)
Stage 4	Deep sleep, brain waves consistently slow (almost all delta)
REM	Breathing becomes more rapid, irregular, shallow; dream state

slower, although they are still punctuated by smaller, faster waves. By stage 4 non-REM sleep, the brain produces extremely slow waves almost exclusively. Stages 3 and 4 are considered deep sleep, during which, ordinarily, it is very difficult to be awakened.

However, this man, a snorer, awakens during stage 2 and stage 4. Is this a case of untreated obstructive sleep apnea (OSA)? It's very likely that it is.

The Incidence of OSA

Epidemiologic surveys show that between 5% and 10% of the middle-aged population has OSA, as defined by more than 10 episodes of OSA per hour of sleep. But most are undetected until a cormobid condition—like this 55-year-old's probable angina—brings them into the health care system, seeking relief.

Chronic obstructive pulmonary disease (COPD), congestive heart failure, cerebrovascular disease, kidney disease and obesity all may underlie the gas exchange disturbances that accompany OSA. As a result, they all are comorbidities commonly seen with this apnea. So are systemic hypertension, pulmonary hypertension, coronary artery disease, nocturnal arrhythmias and stroke. Diabetes, asthma and even emotional stress also are linked to night-time breathing difficulties.

Such comorbid-encompassing pathogenesis is not completely understood, but one key to it appears to be the systemic inflammation that occurs when OSA is present in patients who have such comorbidities—and others, as well. When OSA occurs, it appears to be associated with the same pro-inflammatory forces that are activated in other diseases, as well as the build-up of components essential to plaque formation. All point to an inter-related process that causes expression of adhesion molecules characteristic of other conditions and induction of the atherthosclerotic formation that is consistent with vascular disease.

So far the shared inflammatory process is mostly a matter of speculation. OSA, in some studies, has inflammatory markers that fall after therapy with nocturnal airway pressure. These increases—and plunges—are seen with tumor necrosis factor, interleukin 6, interleukin 8 and C-reactive protein (1). Though the mechanisms are poorly understood, the evidence comes from case-control studies. They don't explain the relationship, but these findings have served to support it in an evidence-based way. For example, levels of interleukin 8, which plays a key role in the process of adhesion of neutrophils and monocytes in the vascular endothelium, show increases in patients with OSA. So is OSA an etiology, an outcome or a co-factor?

The answer is not yet known—but the comorbidities involved are helping clarify a rather murky picture. For example, about one third of patients with systemic hypertension have sleep apnea, while half or more patients with sleep apnea have systemic hypertension. Apart from cardiovascular disease, other disorders, from depression to muscle pain, have a higher prevalence of sleep disturbance—particularly OSA—compared with the general population. A list of associated co-morbid states shows how numerous they are.

Chronic Obstructive Pulmonary Disease (COPD)

Sleep quality is often poor in patients with COPD. Impairment of pulmonary function is associated with decreased total sleep time and efficiency. Sleep can have significant negative effects on respiration in patients with respiratory compromise, resulting in hypoxemia and hypercapnia, which in turn can disturb sleep. Chronic dyspnea and sleep-related hypoxemia likely contribute to the disturbed sleep of patients with COPD. Therefore, therapies such as bronchodilators and nocturnal oxygen supplementation may also improve sleep quality. In addition to lowered pulmonary function and nocturnal oxygen, OSA and other sleep disorders such as insomnia and RLS are common in older patients with COPD and likely contribute to the higher prevalence of sleep complaints in this population.

Diabetes

Sleep disturbances are common among individuals with diabetes. When compared to patients without diabetes, those with diabetes reported higher rates of insomnia and excessive daytime sleepiness. As much as 71% of this population report poor sleep quality. A number of factors contribute to sleep complaints in patients with diabetes. It has been postulated that in patients with type 1 diabetes, rapid changes in glucose levels during sleep cause awakenings and complaints of insomnia. For individuals with type 2 diabetes, sleep disturbances may be related to obesity and obesity-related sleep disorders such as OSA. Sleep-disordered breathing correlates highly with obesity in the population with diabetes. However, independent of obesity, OSA is associated with impaired glucose tolerance, insulin resistance, and hypertension. In addition, there is a correlation between the severity of sleep apnea and of impaired glucose metabolism, insulin resistance, and diabetes.

Other common sources of disturbed sleep in diabetics include chronic discomfort or pain associated with diabetic peripheral neuropathy and restless legs syndrome. Chronic pain, restless legs, and periodic limb movements can cause or exacerbate complaints of difficulty falling asleep and staying asleep. A thorough assessment of sleep quality and treatment of specific sleep disorders, such as sleep apnea and restless legs, can improve the management of metabolic disorders.

Gastrointestinal Disorders

Gastroesophageal reflux disease (GERD), gastritis and peptic-ulcer disease are associated with increased incidences of OSA. The association between OSA, excessive sleepiness and GERD is so well established that the odds of having GERD are known to increase with OSA. The sleep disruption may spur gastric acid secretion, which has a 24-hour cycle that increases acid production in night-time and decreases it early in the day. Thus, such physiologic changes associated with the sleep state, including lying supine, which affects the position of the abdomen and may delay acid clearance by the esophagus, could make an OSA patient more prone to acid reflux at night. In fact, a majority of individuals with chronic GERD report nocturnal heartburn, which could disrupt nocturnal sleep and exacerbate bronchial asthma.

Asthma

Adults with asthma have more complaints of restless sleep and sleepiness than those without asthma, studies show. Sleep can be disrupted by asthma attacks, which occur more frequently in the second half of the night, during REM sleep. The presence of OSA and GERD should also be considered in patients with nocturnal worsening of asthma. Therefore, all patients with asthma should be asked about their sleep quality and examined for symptoms of OSA, which can further disrupt sleep and cause hypoxemia during sleep.

Dementia

Sleep disturbances are very common in patients with dementia and can cause hypersomnolence, irritability, impaired motor and cognitive skills, depression, and fatigue. The underlying pathophysologic mechanism of sleep disturbances in patients with neurodegenerative disorders may involve direct structural alteration of the sleep-wake-generating neurons located in the suprachiasmatic nucleus or may involve external mechanisms such as insufficient light exposure.

In the early part of their disease course, patients with Alzheimer disease commonly present with disruption in sleep-wake rhythmicity, experience increased amounts and frequency of nighttime wakefulness, and have irregular sleep-wake cycles. Later on, they present with a more dramatic reduction of REM sleep, increased REM sleep latency, and alteration of the circadian rhythm, resulting in hypersomnolence. In fact, sleep and cognitive dysfunction are positively correlated in Alzheimer disease.

Chronic Pain and Fibromyalgia

Sleep and pain, the two important vital functions, interact in complex ways that ultimately impact the biologic and behavioral capacity of the individual. Polysomnography studies of patients experiencing acute pain during postoperative recovery demonstrate shortened and fragmented sleep with reduced amounts of REM sleep.

Obesity

Body mass index (BMI) helps confirm OSA. In one study a BMI of at least 25 kg/m^2 had a sensitivity of 93% and a specificity of 74% for OSA. There is currently speculation regarding the association between android-type obesity—fat deposition predominantly in the neck and abdomen—that is commonly associated with metabolic syndrome. This type of obesity is linked to OSA, and the reverse is also true.

Other Influences on OSA

Genetics

A positive family history increases the risk of sleep-disordered breathing (SDB) by twofold to fourfold. First-degree relatives of OSA patients have a 21 to 894% chance of having SDB compared with 10 to 12% of the control subjects. This genetic predisposition is likely to be expressed through craniofacial anatomy that predisposes to OSA, though the genetic predisposition for obesity has also been considered as a potential hereditable pathway to OSA. The craniofacial features which augment risk for OSA include a high and narrow hard palate, and elongated soft palate, small chin, and an abnormal overjet (that is, distance between upper and lower incisive, a dental pattern indicative of abnormal growth pattern of the maxilla, maxilla and mandible, or mandible, and one that may be passed on from parent ot child. There is indication that these anatomical features may become more pronounced as the child grows, if the growth period is punctuated by repetitive bouts of allergies and upper respiratory tract infections, and development of mouth breathing. Mouth breathing may contribute to tonsillar enlargement, a common finding in childhood OSA.

Aging

The geriatric patient population is growing very fast in the United States and around the world. In 2000, 34 million individuals in the United States were older than 65 years. By 2025, this number is expected to go up to 62 million. In light of this fact, geriatricians and other health care providers need to manage an increased number of conditions that increase with aging. Sleep-disordered breathing is one such condition. Elderly patients experience increased sleep fragmentation, decreased sleep efficiency, reduced quality of sleep, and decreased stages 3 and 4. These changes may be related to the underlying age-related neuronal loss, as well as to a disruption of the suprachiasmatic circadian generator.

In addition, these patients often have polypharmacy medication, which has been found to contribute to sleep disorders generally and OSA specifically. In fact, individuals 65 and above are estimated to take 40% or more of all the prescriptions written in the United States and more than half of medications that are sold over the counter. Because age-related changes affect the absorption of these drugs, and because their interaction cause sleep-related side effects, such medications should be investigated for the possible contributory role they play in OSA.

The use of assistive cardiac technology in the elderly also may be present with OSA. In a 2009 study of 98 participating heart patients that was published in *Circulation*, almost 60% of pace-maker patients had undiagnosed sleep apnea.

Moreover, more than one-fifth of the patients had severe sleep apnea, characterized by 30 or more periods of interrupted breathing each hour during sleep. Because of the excessive prevalence of undiagnosed sleep apnea the investigators found, they suggested that all patients referred for a pacemaker should first be screened for sleep apnea.

In the study, researchers investigated the prevalence and consequences of undiagnosed sleep apnea in patients with pacemakers. The patients, with an average age of 64 and undiagnosed with sleep apnea, underwent laboratory monitoring of their sleep: 29 patients had received pacemakers to treat heart failure; 33 patients had a high degree of atrioventricular block; 36 had sinus node disease.

Hormones

Complaints of sleep disturbance are more prevalent among women than men across the entire life span. Alterations in the hormonal environment during the various phases of a woman's life, from menstruation and pregnancy to menopause, likely contribute to insomnia in women.

Among women, there is a sharp rise of approximately 40% in the prevalence of insomnia during the period of transition to menopause and after menopause. Although it is quite clear that sleep quality is decreased with menopause, less is known about the underlying pathophysiology of insomnia in this population. In addition to hormonal changes, hot flushes, depression, anxiety, and sleep disorders such as primary insomnia, restless legs, and sleep apnea have been proposed as causes of sleep disturbance during menopause.

The prevalence of sleep apnea has been found to be higher in both pregnant women and postmenopausal women not on hormone replacement therapy, but lower in pre-menopausal women (3).

The importance of sleep-disordered breathing as an etiology of poor sleep quality in postmenopausal women is now well documented. Menopause is now considered to be an independent risk factor for relatively high AHI.

Stress

Psychological and physiological exposure to stress appears to play a role in OSA, perhaps due to catecholamine release and epinephrine production from the adrenal glands (2). Stress is also related to poorer mental function, due to negative distraction. Such distraction often manifests as worry, which can cause insomnia, frequent awakenings, daytime drowsiness and interruption of the normal circadian rhythms. The disruption of the daily cycle disturbs biorhythms and can cause production of stress hormones known to be related to sleep apnea, such as cortisol.

Substance Abuse

Patients with OSA tend to self-medicate, often with alcohol or drugs, both to fight the depression that often is associated with the disorder, and, possibly, to secure restful sleep. This association with depression seems to play a recurring role in OSA. The overlap between fatigue, stress, depression, sleeping problems and pain has been borne out by workforce studies to determine the most common health complaints for which employees seek treatment. In turn, these are the same conditions that lead to the highest dollar expenditures for employer-backed health plans.

The Burden of OSA

Sleep-disorder breathing is associated with increased risk of all-cause mortality. It affects a substantial number of adults—one in four men and one in 10 women. Further, afflicted individuals are often unaware of having this condition. An increased risk of death has been linked to the effects of OSA on coronary artery disease. And there are other adverse consequences.

In a study of 38 patients who had not been treated for OSA and 20 control participants who were assessed for driving ability after ingesting low-dose alcohol, the OSA group showed far more deviation in steering and had many more collisions during simulated driving than did the control group (4). The authors concluded that OSA probably increased the deleterious effects of alcohol, and they noted that the ill effects of sleep deprivation in this study—as in so many others—led to car crashes. The deficits of OSA are likely to extend to other situations that make people with OSA accident prone, and in some cases, tragically so.

References

1. Ryan S, Taylor C, McNicholas W. Systemic inflammation: a key factor in the pathogenesis of cardiovascular complications in obstructive sleep apnoea sysndrome? *Thorax* 64:631–636, 2009.
2. Drake C, Richardson G, Roehrs T, et al. Vulnerability to stress-related sleep disturbance and hyperarousal. *Sleep* 15;27(2): 285–91, 2004.
3. Bagi K, Malow B. Obstructive sleep apnea—hypopnea syndrome in premenopausal women. In Current Clinical Neurology: Sleep disorders in Women: A Guide to Practical Management. Attarian H. (ed.) Humana Press Inc., Totowa, NJ, 2006.
4. Vakulin A, Baulk S, Catcheside P, et al. Effects of alcohol and sleep restriction on simulated driving performance in untreated patients with obstructive sleep apneas. *Annals of Internal Medicine* 151:447–455, 2009.

CHAPTER 6

Pathophysiology of Obstructive Sleep Apnea

The pathogenesis of obstructive sleep apnea (OSA) and related syndromes, such as central sleep apnea (CSA) and hypopnea, all originate from the same overwhelming abnormalities in respiratory function: not enough air coming from the lungs, not enough space in the throat to assure normal passage of that air, and not enough oxygenation in the blood to maintain normal levels. A pathologic cascade ensues, in which stress hormones are released, inflammatory responses are activated, thrombotic potential is heightened and the risk for ischemia is increased. In general, though, the process begins with a single event—the collapse of the throat, which relaxes and narrows and makes breathing so difficult that snoring is the typical, early outcome and apnea the eventual result.

Pharyngeal Collapse

The capacity of the pharynx to maintain patency during sleep is severely curbed in OSA patients. Normally, the pharynx maintains patency throughout the respiratory cycle during both wakefulness and sleep states, but not in OSA patients. During inspiration, pharyngeal instability occurs, disrupting the balance between the dilating forces generated by muscles and the collapsing force produced by a negative intraluminal pressure, with the latter force becoming dominant. Why does this occur? An association among other cardiovascular conditions is well recognized, though it has not been shown with precision whether this link actually predisposes OSA patients to sleep apnea or simply is related to the changes that that culminate in it. They include atrial fibrillation, hypertension, heart failure and night-time angina. Though OSA is a possible marker for such conditions, and such conditions should prompt investigation of sleep apnea, not all patients with atrial fibrillation, hypertension, heart failure or angina have OSA or CSA.

What is known is that the index of suspicion for any of these conditions should be very high for patients who have sleep difficulties, who are past 50, who are overweight, and who are male. These patients not only have more severe underlying cardiovascular disease than younger patients with OSA usually do, they are more likely to have myocardial infarction. However, younger patients with OSA seem more likely to have hypertension and atrial fibrillation, according to some studies.

It may be that lack of sleep-apnea diagnosis generally accounts for more life-threatening disease in older adults simply because their circulatory systems have been subject to long-acting, apnea-related stressors—hypoxemia, CO_2 retention, oxygen drops—which have prompted vessel remodeling. Apneic stresses are accompanied by surges in sympathetic activity, which, when repetitive, cause serious damage to vessels. Blood pressure levels can reach as high as 240/130 mmHg, a threshold of hemodynamic stress that crosses into severe hypoxemia, hypercapnia, and adrenergic activation. Such activations trigger pathologic processes that inflame tissue, constrict blood vessels, increase heart rate and cause platelet activation, as well as initiating other potentially harmful mechanisms.

Thrombotic Potential

OSA is associated with the production of higher levels of fibrinogen and other serologic components consistent with higher thrombotic risk when elevated. Do these hemostatic mechanisms go awry under sleep apnea-induced changes, leading to chemical production that is tied to a hypercoaguable state? More studies are needed to clarify why high platelet activation occurs and how hypercoaguability specifically is initiated under apneic stress. However, the data so far suggest that this state is a consequence of sleep apnea in some patients.

Endothelial Stress

Sympathetic activation, oxidative stress and inflammation all can arise from repeated episodes of sleep apnea, which in turns selectively impairs small vessels. In obese patients, this selective impairment may be more pronounced, impacting endothelial function even more seriously. Like so many of the processes involved in the pathology of OSA and sleep disturbance, the explanation remains murky as to how triggers to oxidative stress and other possibly deleterious mechanisms of action are ignited. The repetitive hypoxemia and re-oxygenation that is characteristic of OSA during periods of sleep appears to start the chain of events, so that theoretically serves as the triggering action. During this alleged initial phase, some investigations have shown higher levels of barbituric acid reactive substances, as well as increased amounts of isoprostanes and oxidized low-density lipoproproteins.

Glucose Stress

An accumulating body of evidence suggests that sleep deprivation in the presence of OSA goes hand-in-glove with increased catecholamines, which, in turn, promote insulin resistance. The link between glucose intolerance and OSA is so well defined, in fact, that OSA has been suggested as a precursor to the development of insulin resistance.

Such findings have support the relatively long-held findings that changes in the hypothalamic-pituatary-adrenal axis also occur during sleep apnea, increasing cortisol levels. Increased cortisol levels have been demonstrated in the presence of OSA in some patients; Others have failed to find significant escalations of the hormone. One study that aimed to establish definitively the increase in cortisol as a result of sleep apnea failed to find such an association in obese men (1).

The Inflammatory Response

Inflammatory molecules, such as interleukin-6 and C-reactive protein, occur in sleep-deprived OSA patients. There also is evidence of activation of enhanced leukocyte production and chemical processes involved in pro-inflammatory transcription. Theoretically, the OSA episodes induce inflammation despite the reactions that ordinarily suppress it, a capability somehow unleashed by hypoxemia.

Cardiovascular Variability

The sympathetic force incurred by apnea events seems to reduce heart rate variability, according to several studies. Does such lowering of cardiac variability portend increased risk of heart disease? Some studies show it does. Other investigations show that ventricular function is compromised by the intrathoracic pressure changes that occur during OSA, further spurring the possibility of a life-threatening cardiac event. In addition, the vascular endothelial inflammation and enhanced oxidative stress may, in part, explain the accelerated progression of atherosclerosis in patients with OSA (2).

The Mechanisms in OSA in Heart Disease

ST Depression and Myocardial Ischemia

It remains something of a mystery: Why, specifically, does ST depression occur during OSA? Do vascular impediments, such as the sympathetic-driven vasoconstriction that has been previously described, cause this? Is it due to the recurrent hypoxemia? Do the rather dramatic changes in intrathoracic and cardiac transmural pressures impact ST depression?

It appears from studies on patients with sleep apnea and coronary artery disease that not only is ST depression common, so is ischemia—and eventually infarction among patients who are not treated for severe sleep apnea. More than half of sudden death from cardiac-related events in OSA happen during sleep hours, in dramatic contrast to the traditional early-morning "window of variability" of 6 am to 11 am for most people who die from heart attack. In addition, the likelihood of myocardial infarction in patients with OSA increases according to disease severity.

In hypoxia, biological responses are initiated that, in turn, trigger other cellular activities damaging to tissue. It is well established that myocardial infarction, stroke and venous thromboembolism all occur in the presence of oxygen deprivation. Mediators of this may be muted in the presence of hypoxia; Hypoxia may stimulate or generate actions that suppress oxygen. The master regulator elicited by hypoxia is not fully understood, but it is known to cause tissue stress. Investigators have looked at this relationship and found evidence of involvement by the receptor for advanced glycation end products (3).

Renal Disease
Although traditionally OSA has been linked to heart disease, increasingly it has been documented in end-stage renal disease. The etiologic reason is believed to be a two-step cause and effect: Induction of blood pressure and sympathetic nerve discharge occurs, which damages the vascular beds.

The symptoms of sleep apnea in kidney patients are typical. They often have excessive daytime drowsiness, which is very typically a physical sign of possible OSA. However, the pattern of OSA may be distinctive. Unlike many other patient groups, they tend to have a mixed incidence of both OSA and CSA.

Pulmonary Arterial Hypertension
Hypoxemia is known to induce this form of hypertension by increasing pulmonary arterial pressure during lapses in sleeping. Thus, there are frequent episodes of pulmonary arterial pressure during sleep, but there may be no obvious such obvious episoces in the day time. It has not been elucidated, or at least not elucidated fully, whether CPAP provides sustained prevention or reduction of arterial hypertension in these patients. However, investigations so far show fairly definitive short-term benefit.

Snore Development and Atherosclerosis
OSA is linked to heavy snoring, and heavy snoring is linked to OSA. However, previously the link to atherosclerosis was only

strongly implied—not etiologically proven. Now there is growing evidence that heavy snoring is independently related to the risk to developing carotid artery atherosclerosis.

Recently, Australian researchers, noting vascular risk factors seem to be higher in snorers, evaluated 110 volunteers—a group divided between those who snored and those who didn't—to determine if snoring might predispose cardiovascular disease. They assessed ultrasound scans of carotid and femoral arteries in study participants, as well as polysomnograms from sleep studies. Their findings show that heavy snoring that seems to be free of OSA actually often includes mild, non-hypoxic events. They also found that heavy snoring was significantly associated with carotid atherosclerosis.

Based on these results, the investigators concluded that heavy snoring significantly increases the risk of carotid atherosclerosis, and, as a result of this increased risk, also heightens the probability of stroke. In fact, they found the increase to be independent of other risk factors, including measures of nocturnal hypoxia and OSA severity. They concluded that the high prevalence of snoring constitutes as substantial public health concern, in terms of carotid atherosclerosis and the risk of stroke (4).

References

1. Dadoun F, Darmon P, Achard V, et al. Effect of sleep apnea syndrome on the circadian profile of cortisol in obese men. *Am J Physiol Endocrinol Metab* 293:E466–E474, 2007.
2. Jelic S and Le Jemtel T. Inflammation, oxidative stress, and the vascular endothelium in obstructive sleep apnea. *Trends in Cardiovascular Med* 18:253–260, 2008.
3. Chang J, Wendt T, Qu W, et al. Oxygen deprivation triggers upregulation fo early growth response-1 by the receptor for advanced glycation end products. *Circ Res.* 102:905–913, 2008.
4. Lee S, Amis T, Byth K, et al. Heavy snoring as a cause of carotid artery atherosclerosis. *Sleep* 31(9):1207–1213, 2008.

CHAPTER 7

Treatment of Sleep Apnea

Evidence is mounting that obstructive sleep apnea (OSA) is independently related to many cardiovascular disorders, including hypertension, coronary artery disease, cerebrovascular disease and congestive heart disease (CHF). CHF has been linked to central sleep apnea (CSA), as well. Treatment strategies for both have been suggested to be potentially life-saving, although such declarative pronouncements are complicated by the fact that the two syndromes seem to be multifactorial, and they are confounded by other common disease states, such as obesity. As a result, there is debate about how strong the risk factor of sleep apnea truly independently relates to the development of heart disease, and which approaches to treatment of OSA and CSA may the most scientifically valid in light of that risk, particularly when patient quality-of-life issues are taken into consideration.

Options for CSA Treatment

There is no consensus about how CSA should be treated, and there is no compelling evidence that treating it reduces mortality. There is, however, research showing that treatment can lower the apnea-hypopnea index (AHI), reduce sleep fragmentation and lessen daytime sleepiness. Two approaches have succeeded in doing just that: Use of angiotensin-converting enzyme has been shown to reduce AHI and desaturation in patients with mild-to-moderate heart failure: Nocturnal oxygen has been shown to eradicate apnea-related hypoxia. But neither has been proven to improve cardiac function or long-term quality of life.

Another agent is theophylline, which has been demonstrated to reduce CSA, but the drug is not showing a positive impact on any of the clinical variables, such as right or left ejection fraction. Moreover, since it is pro-arrhythmic, it is not recommended for CSA reduction.

CPAP and bilevel PAP have shown promise for CSA, and they remain a focus of possible "best-practice" treatment, but the results using either one have not been universally successful at addressing CSA alone in CHF patients. Both therapies have been linked to significant improvement in ejection fraction and more restful sleep. However, neither has been shown to change the course of the disease in CHF patients nor to prevent or shorten hospital length-of-stays associated with the condition.

A role for cardiac resynchronization therapy also has been suggested—early trials show it can be used to attenuate CSA—but the results have been from small, non-randomized patient groups and more studies are needed to confirm a significant benefit. In contrast, the treatment of OSA by positive airway pressure has become a mainstay: A clearer clinical benefit is derived from it. Because CSA and OSA are so frequently concurrent, a more distinct therapeutic picture may emerge for CSA as OSA continues to attract some fairly intense research for improving positive air delivery.

Positive Airway Pressure Treatment for OSA

Continuous positive airway pressure (CPAP) restores stability to respiration by delivering nearly constant positive pressure during both inspiration and exhalation. In contrast, bilevel positive airway pressure, bilevel PAP, exerts two different pressures: A higher one during inspiration; a lower one for exhalation. Both CPAP and bilevel PAP provide fixed-level pressures, which necessitate finding an optimal pressure for night-time sleep, then relying on those measures. Bilevel PAP is applied by setting the inspiratory pressure to a higher pressure than the expiratory pressure. Therefore, the gradient for flow is determined by the difference between inspiratory and expiratory pressures. Hence the resistance of the airways, combined with patient effort, drives the volume of inspiration. Both positive airway-pressure methods have been shown to significantly improve quality of life compared with sham CPAP groups in random case-control studies.

This has been borne out by clinical observation, as well by the patients themselves and the opinions of family members and friends of patients who have undergone treatment (1). But sleep position, sleep stages and even body temperature all change during the night, making the capacity to change pressures desirable, too.

Research has shown higher pressure typically is needed during REM sleep, when the supine position is assumed, and higher pressure also may be warranted during nasal congestion.

Nor is sleep the quiescent state most people assume: Blankets may get pulled on or tossed off, the dream state may get acted upon with flailing limbs, and body position changes every few minutes in people who have a more restless pattern of sleep. All of these can jostle and impact the PAP system, sometimes without the patient even being aware of it. Though CPAP and bilevel PAP have proven extremely beneficial in helping many OSA patients get a good night's sleep, over and again, the method has not proven a universal panacea to OSA—many potential side effects have been documented, side affects that can severely curtail adherence.

Side Effects of Positive Airway Pressure Systems

Intolerance of the mask is one of the most common reasons for non-compliance. Mask leaks that allow air to escape, sometimes blowing onto the face and into the eyes are a major reason for discontinuation of use. Bruises are another. Tightening head straps to help the mask stay in place can result in abrasions.

Also, the masks require upkeep—cleaning and replacement—that may cause patients to view the system as a chore. Complaints from users include observations such as: "It is an uncomfortable fit" and "I can't change positions without the mask coming ajar," a reference to the seal being broken during movement. Mouth leaks also can cause dryness, which, in turn, can incite awakening—this wakefulness often is the very thing the patient is seeking to avoid, and may have been the reason treatment was sought in the first place. As a result, adherence continues to be challenge in using positive airway pressure.

But there is reason for optimism. Now, more flexible materials for the mask and hose have increased the comfort of CPAP technology. Construction of the masking component continues to evolve, and many systems now expand, balloon-like, against the face under pressure. Seal breakage also is easier to prevent, thanks to the development of nasal prongs that add a tiny "pillow" structure helps keep the system sealed at the nasal bridge, even under the strain of night-time tossing and turning. Because nasal symptoms, such as congestion and rhinorrhea, can arise and persist with the use of CPAP or bilevel PAP, heated humidification is included in some treatment plans. Nasal steroids, non-sedating anti-histamines and decongestants before bedtime all have been suggested as alternatives for nasal problems related to positive airway pressure.

Noise from the process itself—the blower attachment and the air stream that exits the mask—can be another deterrent. New designs that make the system quieter address this auditory effect, although it can still perturb a user or bed partner who is bothered by night-time noises. Some systems have mitigated this problem by making the sound not only softer but rhythmic, in an attempt to mimic white-noise machines that promote sleep for some people. Some users also experience a sense of claustrophobia from the device, but repeated utilization or, as it is sometimes called, "CPAP adaptation," may abolish this feeling. If there seem to be psychological barriers to CPAP acceptance—expressed feelings of entrapment by the device, or excessive worry about relying on it—counseling often can help alleviate the resistance. In some cases, contact with an experienced user, a support group or trained counselor can reduce the anxiety and reluctance.

Education about OSA and CPAP is now routine at many centers, including "PAP clinics" where patients are acquainted with the purpose of the technology they are about to undertake. Such programs have been shown to boost adherence, as do follow-up phone calls or other forms of contact from health care providers. A significant portion of such patient education can be performed by nurses, office staff and respiratory therapists, but adherence is better when a physician is involved in that process, too, studies show.

One reason that physician involvement appears to have an adherence-boosting effect is that the benefits of treatment can be affirmed during a doctor-patient encounter, where the potential for disease-risk reversal can be explained. Reductions of systemic and pulmonary arterial pressures are well documented during the administration of positive airway pressure, and the method has been shown to prevent apnea, hypopnea, and escalations of blood pressure that persist during the day. In fact, some research has shown that CPAP significantly reduces the risk of coronary heart disease and stroke.

As has been observed in the medical literature, a positive attitude on the part of the health care provider—not just the patient—is a key to adherence. "If the health care provider appears unconvinced of the merits of positive airway pressure, the patient is unlikely to be a believer, and is, therefore, a poor risk for successful home therapy," advises one guide to the therapy published by sleep-medicine specialists.

Pharmacologic Treatment

Protiptyline has been shown to be partly effective for treating mild OSA, but the trials have been small and improvement in daytime somnolence and nocturnal oxygenation lack long-term follow-up. Protriptylline apparently acts to decrease REM sleep while stabilizes upper-airway passages. Fluoxetine has been shown to accomplish similar results, with fewer side effects. Paroxetine has resulted in a modest decrease in the AHI during non-REM sleep, so that selective serotonin re-uptake inhibitor may hold promise. A study of OSA in canines found that medroxyprogesterone acetate induces hyperventilation. Other studies on it indicate it may be useful for patients with obesity-hypoventilation syndrome, lower PCO_2 and reduce AHI. However, such results have been mixed and side effects such as thromboembolism make it contraindicated for some patients.

Modafinil has been used to reduce daytime drowsiness in OSA but such a use is experimental and, in general practice, is not recommended.

Overview of Surgical Procedures

Tracheotomy

Tracheotomy remains a standard surgical treatment for OSA. It is different from all other surgical procedures for OSA because it doesn't involve any of the upper airways. It has achieved levels of success that are higher than any other procedures. But is unpopular with patients, and therefore is now performed only in those with severe OSA who have failed other treatments, including CPAP, bilevel PAP or other methods.

Nasal Reconstruction

Nasal obstruction or lack of patency has been implicated in increased oral breathing and mouth opening during sleep. Airway obstruction occurs due to the rotation of the mandible and the migration of the tongue bas back into the pharynx; This situation can also inhibit optimal use of positive airway pressure. To determine whether patency is compromised, examination should be done of the nose in the alar cartilage and nasal valve region, at the septum, and in the turbinates.

The use of temperature-controlled radiofrequency energy to reduce hypertrophic turbinates is showing promise as a technique for improving the capability of CPAP flow.

Oropharyngeal Surgery
Uvulopalatopharyngoplasty

This surgery, which is performed under general anesthesia, removes part of the soft palate, uvula, and a portion of the lateral pharynegeal wall. Tonsillar tissue, if present, also is taken out. This addresses the oropharyngeal obstruction; its success rate is only approximately 40%.

Uvulopalatal Flap
This approach modifies uvulopharyngoplasty, and involves the retraction of the uvula, superiorly, toward the hard-soft palate junction, following a limited removal of the uvula, lateral pharyngeal wall, and mucosa. This widens the oropharyngeal airway and often reduces the potential for post-surgical complications.

Laser-assisted Uvulopalatoplasty
This approach, which was introduced as an office-based procedure for the treatment of snoring, involves removal of the uvula and a part of the soft palate by CO_2 laser incisions and vaporization. It amputates most of the uvula, incises and vaporizes part of the soft palate. The laser also can be used to vaporize mucosal or tonsil tissue, if that is needed. This method has not had long-term follow-up and some medical groups believe there are insufficient data to recommend it for the treatment of OSA.

Hypopharyngeal Surgery
Genioglossus Advancement
Genioglossus advancement, a technique that targets the tongue, was the first procedure to specifically address obstruction by this structure. The surgical approach is based on the fact that many cases of OSA show decreased posterior airway space and increased distance between the mandible and the hyoid. After surgery, these measurements have been shown to improve, and that improvement has been confirmed by post-surgery polysomnography.

Does the genioglossus muscle play a critical role in nocturnal airway obstruction? An improved incorporation of the genioglossus muscle in the advanced portion of the mandible seems to set the stage for more regular respiration. The surgery is advanced, does not alter the shape of the mandible, but transfers tension to the tongue musculature, reducing the posterior displacement that has been occurring during sleep. The procedure is performed inside the oral cavity, with an incision in the mucosa made just below the mucogingival junction; A subperiosteal flap is reflected, exposing the anterior mandible and mental nerves. Finger palpation of the genial tubercle and genioglossus muscle can pinpoint these structures on the floor of the mouth with the aid of the lateral cephalometric radiograph. Osteotomy in the shape of a rectangle is made to incorporate the geniotubercle; The geniotubercle is moved forward, and partly rotated, to forestall retraction back into the floor of the mouth.

Hyoid Advancement

Anatomically, the hyoid complex is a crucial part of the hypopharynx. The posterior airway space appears to be strongly influenced by it. So there is scientifically sound reason to believe that surgical intervention at the hyoid level improves the hypopharyngeal airway. However, some hypopharyngeal OSA is resolved with only genioglossus advancement, so hyoid advancement may not always be necessary. As a result, hyoid advancement often is a separate surgery that follows genioglossus advancement when necessary. The technique involves suspension of the hyoid to the superior thyroid cartilage; This improves the hypopharyngeal airway but is less invasive than previous techniques.

A horizontal incision is made above the hyoid bone, inferiorly along the suprahyoid musculature of the hyoid structure, and infra-hyoid muscles are removed from the body of the hyoid, isolating it. The suprahyoid muscles are left intact.

Maxillomandibular Advancement

Maxillofacial abnormality often is found in patients with OSA. The abnormality enlarges the pharyngeal and hypopharyngeal airway by physically expanding the skeletal framework, causing collapse of the suprahyoid and pharynx muscles, as well as pharyngeal-wall collapse.

This surgery can be performed as the initial one, or performed after all other procedures have failed to sufficiently improve OSA. Other surgical approaches are less invasive but some patients, particularly those who have either severe sleep apnea or significant maxillomandibular deformity, may perefer this as a frontline treatment.

Maxillomandibular Expansion

Expansion of the maxilla and mandible for the treatment of OSA shows promising results but a paucity of data so far. A small series of patients who have undergone it show improved mean AHI indices and improvement of the mean lowest oxygen saturation at more than a year of follow-up.

Temperature-Controlled Radiofrequency Tongue-Based Reduction

Therapeutic ablation of tissue to reduce the tongue base had been studied prospectively in small numbers of patients. In one series, respiration difficulties improved substantially and complications were minimal. No changes in speech or swallowing occurred. Complications included minor tongue ulceration that spontaneously healed, pain during swallowing that stopped after several weeks, and an abscess formation requiring drainage of the site on the tongue. Other investigators have confirmed the benefits of radiofrequency for treatment of OSA. However, the use of it by itself is usually not successful for completely managing OSA. Also, there can in some patients be a relapse of OSA. Thus, RF is frequently used adjunctively, often along with other surgical approaches.

Surgical Management of Patients

A majority of the patients with OSA require surgical intervention at the oropharyngeal and hypopharyngeal levels. It is curative for most—a surgical result that is comparable to that found with nasal CPAP. However, these patients obviously undergo invasive procedures to achieve results, a situation that carries special risk and necessitates caution and care.

Pre-operative Period

If a patient can use CPAP, it needs to be undertaken shortly prior to surgery in order to reverse sleep debt prior to the procedure.

Otherwise, REM "rebound" can occur in the postoperative period. Among patients who have a difficult airway—those with significant obesity, increased neck circumference (>46 cm), or associated skeletal deformities such as mandibular deficiency and low hyoid bone—fiber-optic intubation while awake or tracheotomy bears careful consideration. There have been concerns in the medical community over treating OSA in very obese individuals both because of risk from surgery in this patient group and the suspicion that treating OSA has little impact since the effect of therapy is overwhelmed by the complications of obesity itself (2).

Peri-operative Period

Extreme caution is necessary for the use of narcotics after general anesthesia in OSA patients with postoperative airway edema. Certain medications promote sleep apnea. Before discharge, patients need to be educated about the risk of prescription drug use and alcohol ingestion, because adequate pain control is essential to a satisfactory recovery period but narcotic use poses risks. Nasal CPAP with humidified oxygen for two weeks following discharge can promote healing in patients who ordinarily cannot tolerate nasal CPAP.

Conclusion

There is overwhelming evidence that OSA adversely affects quality of life and well being. And, although nasal CPAP can be an effective treatment for the majority of patients, it is very much limited by patient adherence. Even among motivated patients, the effectiveness may never reach ideal levels. Surgical therapy is still viewed as an alternative in patients who are intolerant of positive airway pressure but surgery has been proven to be highly successful in the management of OSA. By using a logical and stepwise protocol, the outcome for OSA can be improved and the complications form surgery minimized or avoided.

Mean hospital stay varies, but in general is about two days. Complications associated with genioglossus advancement and hyoid suspension are infection, injury of tooth roots requiring root canal therapy, permanent paresthesia and anesthesia of the mandibular incisors, and seroma. The risk of major complications, such as mandibular fracture, alteration of speech, or alteration of swallow or aspiration has not been documented in tertiary care setting with experienced surgeons.

References

1. Verster J, Pandi-Perumal S, Streiner D (eds.). Sleep and quality of life in clinical medicine. Humana Press, Totowa, NJ, 2008.
2. Pack A, Gislason T. Obstructive sleep apnea and cardiovascular disease: a perspective and future directions. *Prog Cardiovasc Dis* 51(5): 434–451, 2009.